THE THYROID DIET COOKBOOK FOR BEGINNERS

Learn About Essential Nutrients And Ingredients Crucial For Thyroid Health. Empower Yourself With Knowledge To Optimize Your Diet And Well-Being

JESSICA C. STEPHEN

Disclaimer

The information in this book is meant solely for educational reasons. This book's contents are not meant to be used in place of expert medical advice, diagnosis, or treatment. Any decisions you make about your health must be discussed with a licensed healthcare provider.

Every effort has been made by the author to guarantee that the material in this book is correct and current as of the date of publication. Still, since medical knowledge advances rapidly, new studies might be conducted that change our understanding this illness and how best to manage it with food.

This book may contains references to and mentions of various people, things, websites, organizations, and other entities that the author does not support, advocate, or have any association with. There is no implied sponsorship or collaboration; all references and remarks are made only for informational purposes.

In order to address their individual health concerns, readers are advised to independently verify any information contained in this book and to consult with healthcare specialists. Any negative effects arising from the use or implementation of the material in this book, whether direct or indirect, are not the responsibility of the author or the publisher.

The dietary suggestions and counsel provided in this book are broad in scope and might not be appropriate for every individual. Readers are recommended to seek tailored counsel from trained healthcare specialists as individual health problems and demands differ.

The reader accepts the conditions of this disclaimer by reading this book.

About This Book

"The Thyroid Health Diet cookbook" is an invaluable resource for anyone looking to maximize thyroid function with a holistic approach that incorporates lifestyle, diet, and doable meal planning. The first section of this book provides readers with a comprehensive overview of thyroid health, including an explanation of the thyroid gland and typical illnesses that are related to it. This background information prepares the reader for an examination of the critical role that diet plays in maintaining thyroid function.

This book's examination of substances that stimulate the thyroid is one of its strongest points. It explores important vitamins and minerals, antioxidants, and omega-3 fatty acids, offering a comprehensive knowledge of their roles in thyroid function. Readers are further empowered to make educated dietary decisions by the emphasis on picking items that actively promote thyroid function or by being aware of those that may impede it.

This tutorial focuses mostly on meal planning, including a section that deconstructs the art of creating well-balanced meals. This book gains a concrete, useful dimension with the addition of sample meal plans for increasing thyroid function and useful advice for meal preparation and batch cooking. The focus on meals designed to promote thyroid function during breakfast, lunches, and dinners takes into account the daily obstacles people may have in adhering to a thyroid-healthy diet.

This book goes beyond recipes to provide side dishes, snacks, and drinks that are specially made to support thyroid function. The author offers a wide range of solutions to suit different dietary needs and preferences, from guilt-free sweets to nutrient-dense side dishes. Recipes for special occasions provide a thoughtful touch and help people navigate social situations while keeping their thyroid health in mind.

This book acknowledges the role that lifestyle choices and exercise have in thyroid health in addition to nutrition. Readers are provided with a comprehensive grasp of the lifestyle elements that contribute to thyroid health overall by exploring stress management approaches, the significance of physical activity, and the impact of sleep on thyroid function.

One particularly noteworthy element is the 30-day food plan that boosts thyroid function. It includes shopping lists, preparation advice, and week-by-week meal planning. This doable road plan provides a crucial layer of structure and accountability, along with instructions on monitoring advancement and making required modifications.

To sum up, "The Thyroid Health diet cookbook" is it's an all-inclusive guide that enables people to take control of their thyroid health by making educated dietary and lifestyle decisions. This book is a vital resource for anyone trying to promote healthy thyroid function and general well-being because of its abundance of knowledge, helpful advice, and variety of recipes.

Table of Contents

CHAPTER 1

OVERVIEW OF THYROID HEALTH

Knowledge Of The Thyroid Gland

The thyroid gland is a butterfly-shaped organ in the neck that is essential for controlling the body's many metabolic processes. It is a component of the endocrine system and generates the hormones triiodothyronine (T3) and thyroxine (T4), which affect how quickly cells use nutrients to make energy. The delicate regulation of these hormones is necessary to preserve the general equilibrium of the organism. Through the secretion of thyroid-stimulating hormone (TSH), the pituitary gland carefully regulates thyroid function, maintaining a precise balance.

This balance is frequently upset by thyroid diseases. Weak hormone production by the thyroid causes hypothyroidism, which manifests as symptoms like weight gain, lethargy, and cold intolerance. On the other hand, symptoms of hyperthyroidism, which include increased heart rate, heat intolerance, and weight loss, are brought on by an overactive thyroid. Comprehending the complex feedback mechanisms associated with thyroid regulation is vital to appreciate the range of illnesses that may impact this essential gland.

Typical Thyroid Conditions

The function of the thyroid gland can be impacted by several thyroid conditions, each having unique traits and symptoms. The most common disorder, hypothyroidism, is frequently brought on by autoimmune diseases such as iodine deficiency or Hashimoto's thyroiditis. Underproduction of thyroid hormones causes a slow metabolism, which in turn causes weariness, weight gain, and cognitive decline.

On the other hand, an overactive thyroid that overproduces hormones is known as hyperthyroidism, and it is frequently brought on by illnesses like Graves' disease. This results in symptoms including anxiety, elevated heart rate, and weight loss. Thyroid nodules are growths on the thyroid that can either be malignant or benign. Given that untreated thyroid diseases can have far-reaching repercussions on the body, knowledge of these disorders is crucial for prompt diagnosis and efficient treatment.

Nutrition's Function in Thyroid Health

Sustaining adequate thyroid function is largely dependent on nutrition. Thyroid hormones require the trace element iodine as one of their constituents. Hypothyroidism can result from insufficient iodine intake, which highlights the need to consume iodine-rich foods including dairy products, seafood, and seaweed in the diet.

Due to its role in the transformation of T4 into the more active T3 hormone, selenium is another essential vitamin for thyroid health. Including foods high in selenium, such as seafood, sunflower seeds, and Brazil nuts, can help promote thyroid function. Furthermore, optimal metabolic health depends on a diet that is well-balanced and contains enough of various vitamins and minerals, such as zinc and vitamin D.

But when ingested in excess, some foods—known as goitrogens—can interfere with thyroid function. Among these are cruciferous foods, such as cabbage and broccoli. The effects of these meals on thyroid function can be lessened by cooking them.

In summary, a thorough grasp of the thyroid gland, prevalent thyroid problems, and the role that nutrition plays in thyroid health offers a solid basis for preserving and advancing general health. People can choose a healthy lifestyle to support a functioning thyroid by being aware of the delicate hormonal balance and the influence of nutrition on thyroid function.

CHAPTER 2

THYROID-SUPPORTING FOODS

<u>Vital Minerals And Vitamins For Healthy Thyroid Function</u>

Ensuring a sufficient intake of vital vitamins and minerals is paramount in sustaining thyroid function, which is critical for maintaining overall health. Iodine and selenium are two of the most important of these. Triiodothyronine (T3) and thyroxine (T4), the two thyroid hormones, are fundamentally made of iodine. Hypothyroidism is a disorder characterized by an underactive thyroid caused by an iodine shortage. Conversely, selenium plays a crucial role in the transformation of T4 into the more potent T3 form, which supports the ideal activity of the thyroid.

Vitamin D is also necessary for thyroid function. It helps control thyroid function and affects the immunological system. Another essential vitamin that helps the thyroid function is vitamin A, which does this by encouraging the synthesis of thyroxine. Thyroid hormone-related metabolic activities are among the many metabolic processes that the B vitamins, especially B2, B3, and B6, are engaged in. It's essential to make sure you have enough of these vitamins if you want to keep your thyroid healthy.

Antioxidants to Support the Thyroid

Strong substances called antioxidants fight oxidative stress, a condition connected to thyroid dysfunction. Because of its high metabolic activity and exposure to reactive oxygen species, the thyroid is vulnerable to oxidative injury. Strong antioxidants like vitamins C and E, as well as minerals like copper and zinc, shield the thyroid from oxidative damage.

Fruits and vegetables high in vitamin C help protect thyroid cells from harm by scavenging free radicals. Nuts and seeds are rich sources of vitamin E, which protects the thyroid by halting lipid peroxidation. Zinc is a trace element that is essential to antioxidant enzyme systems and thyroid cell structural integrity. When combined with zinc, copper helps shield the thyroid gland from oxidative stress.

By reducing oxidative stress, eating a range of foods high in antioxidants, such as berries, nuts, seeds, and colorful vegetables, can support a healthy thyroid.

The Thyroid and Omega-3 Fatty Acids

Walnuts, flaxseeds, and fatty fish are the main sources of omega-3 fatty acids, which are essential for maintaining thyroid function. Thyroid health benefits from the anti-inflammatory qualities of EPA (eicosapentaenoic acid) and DHA (docosahexaenoic acid), the two primary forms of omega-3 fatty acids.

Omega-3 fatty acids assist in preventing thyroid function impairment caused by chronic inflammation by encouraging a healthy immune response and decreasing inflammation. To support appropriate cellular function, these fatty acids also contribute to the construction of cell membranes, including those of thyroid cells.

Furthermore, omega-3s improve the bloodstream's ability to carry thyroid hormones efficiently, which guarantees that the hormones will reach their target regions and start working. Including foods high in omega-3s in the diet or taking supplements can be helpful tactics to support thyroid health in general.

To sum up, following the recommendations for important vitamins and minerals, adding antioxidants, and making sure you get enough omega-3 fatty acids will help you keep your thyroid functioning properly. People can take charge of their thyroid health and general well-being by eating a nutrient-rich diet that supports thyroid function.

CHAPTER 3

SELECTING FOODS GOOD FOR THE THYROID

Foods To Promote Healthy Thyroid Function

Certain meals are essential for maintaining good thyroid function when it comes to thyroid health. Foods high in iodine are essential among them since iodine is a crucial part of thyroid hormones. Prominent sources of iodine include seafood, dairy products, and iodized salt. Including these in one's diet guarantees that the thyroid obtains the components it needs to manufacture hormones.

Moreover, selenium is yet another vital mineral that supports thyroid function. Enzymes involved in the conversion of thyroid hormones require selenium as a cofactor. Fish, sunflower seeds, and Brazil nuts are all great sources of selenium. People can improve the effectiveness of thyroid hormone synthesis and metabolism by consuming these foods.

The thyroid depends on vitamins, especially vitamin D. Sufficient amounts of vitamin D aid in thyroid hormone regulation and immune system support. Getting enough vitamin D can be achieved by fatty fish, fortified dairy products, and sun exposure. The delicate balance of thyroid hormones in the body depends on the synergy of these nutrients.

Additionally, iron, zinc, and omega-3 fatty acids support thyroid function. Iron is necessary for the creation of thyroid hormones, zinc aids in their conversion, and omega-3 fatty acids contribute to the reduction of inflammation and the maintenance of a healthy thyroid environment. You can include foods like nuts, beans, fatty fish, and lean meats in your diet to help your thyroid.

To sum up, a diet high in vitamins, zinc, iron, iodine, selenium, and omega-3 fatty acids provides a strong basis for maintaining thyroid function. The interaction of these nutrients guarantees the thyroid gland's normal operation, which enhances general health.

Items To Limit Or Steer Clear Of For Healthy Thyroid

When aiming for thyroid wellness, it's important to be aware of which foods can interfere with thyroid function, even as certain foods promote thyroid health. Broccoli, cabbage, and Brussels sprouts are examples of cruciferous vegetables.

These plants contain substances called goitrogens, which can disrupt the production of thyroid hormones. Cooking these veggies can lessen their goitrogenic effects, although moderation is important for those who have thyroid issues.

Consuming too many soy products might also be harmful. Thyroid hormone absorption may be inhibited by substances found in soy. While it's generally thought that consuming soy in moderation is harmless, people who have thyroid problems may need to watch how much they eat.

Thyroid function may be adversely affected by highly processed diets, particularly those that contain unhealthy fats and refined carbohydrates, which can exacerbate inflammation. These meals have the potential to worsen underlying thyroid disorders and upset the hormonal balance.

Consuming too much caffeine may hinder the absorption of thyroid hormones. Although most people can take moderate doses of caffeine, excessive use is not recommended, particularly for those who have thyroid issues.

To sum up, limiting caffeine, avoiding processed foods, reducing soy intake, and being aware of goitrogenic veggies are all essential for preserving thyroid function. People can more effectively control and maintain their thyroid function by eating well-informedly.

The Value of Well-Balanced Diet:

A healthy, well-balanced diet is essential for general well-being, and its importance is even more so when considering thyroid function. Numerous nutrients are necessary for the thyroid gland to operate properly, and eating a balanced diet makes sure that these vital components are always available.

A well-balanced diet helps the body's complex hormonal dance, which keeps the thyroid and other glands functioning in harmony. Sufficient consumption of vitamins, minerals, and macronutrients gives the thyroid the resources it needs to efficiently synthesize and regulate hormones.

Additionally, maintaining a healthy weight is beneficial for those who have thyroid issues. A balanced diet aids in reaching and maintaining a healthy weight. Both hypothyroidism and hyperthyroidism can have an impact on weight. Consequently, this enhances the general metabolic equilibrium and energy reserves.

A varied and well-balanced diet also supports the gut microbiome's health. A healthy microbiome has a good impact on the conversion and usage of thyroid hormones, and the gut plays a part in the absorption of nutrients. Consuming meals high in fiber, probiotics, and prebiotics helps maintain gut health, which in turn helps thyroid function.

In addition to directly supporting thyroid function, a diet high in a variety of nutrients also helps maintain overall hormonal and metabolic balance. A balanced diet should be prioritized by people to prevent thyroid problems and maintain good thyroid function.

CHAPTER 4

MEAL PREPARATION FOR HEALTHY THYROIDS

Creating Balanced Meals to Maintain Thyroid Health

The formulation of well-balanced meals is an essential component of supporting thyroid health, which is directly linked to general well-being. You can be sure that your body is getting all the nutrients it needs to keep your thyroid functioning at its best with a balanced diet. It's critical to incorporate a range of nutrient-dense foods while creating meals for thyroid health.

Prioritize including a variety of macronutrients, such as proteins, carbs, and fats. Lean meats, seafood, beans, and legumes are good sources of protein, which is important for thyroid hormone production. Whole grains, fruits, and vegetables include complex carbs, which help control blood sugar levels and deliver energy gradually.

Nuts, avocados, and olive oil are good sources of fat that aid in the generation and absorption of hormones.

Incorporate a variety of micronutrients as well, especially those that are essential for thyroid function. A vital mineral for thyroid function, iodine is present in dairy products, seafood, and seaweed. Seafood, nuts, and seeds are rich sources of selenium, which aids in the conversion of thyroid hormones. Meat, nuts, and seeds are good sources of zinc, which is needed for the generation of thyroid hormone. Thyroid function is also supported by ensuring a sufficient diet of vitamins, such as A, D, and B vitamins.

Taking into account a food's glycemic index is another aspect of meal planning. Choose low-glycemic foods to avoid blood sugar surges, which can affect thyroid function. Nutrients for optimal thyroid health can be found in a well-rounded dish that includes healthy grains, lean proteins, and a rainbow of veggies.

Example Menus For Thyroid-Boosting Foods

The food content and portion sizes must be carefully considered while creating sample meal plans for thyroid health. You can incorporate a range of foods that promote thyroid function in your daily meal plan.

Think about having a bowl of oatmeal with berries and chia seeds on top for breakfast. Berries supply fiber and antioxidants, whereas oats offer complex carbohydrates.

Omega-3 fatty acids are included in chia seeds and are essential for thyroid function.

A grilled chicken salad with a variety of vibrant vegetables might be the meal. Vital vitamins are found in leafy greens, while thyroid hormone production is supported by the lean protein in chicken. Richness is added to the salad by incorporating an avocado or other healthy fat source.

Steamed broccoli and quinoa might accompany baked salmon, which is high in omega-3s and selenium. Broccoli adds vitamins and minerals necessary for thyroid health, while quinoa offers a complete protein.

A handful of mixed nuts can provide zinc and selenium, while Greek yogurt with honey on top can provide probiotics and iodine.

Advice for Batch Cooking and Meal Preparation

While leading a hectic lifestyle, effective meal preparation and bulk cooking are essential for maintaining a thyroid-friendly diet. Making a plan in advance guarantees that nutrient-dense meals are available and also saves time.

Make a weekly meal plan first, selecting meals that support thyroid health. Making bigger batches of food that can be portioned and frozen for later use is known as batch cooking. Think about prepping veggies, grains, and proteins in large quantities to make it simple to put together a variety of meals throughout the week.

Get high-quality storage containers to preserve the freshness of prepared meals. Managing freshness and reducing food waste can be achieved by dating and labeling containers.

To avoid boredom, mix up your batch-cooked meals by adding different flavors and textures. To make meals interesting and filling, switch up your protein sources, use new herbs and spices, and add different veggies.

Foods that are easily reheated without sacrificing flavor and texture should be given priority. Batch cooking works well for soups, stews, and casseroles because their tastes tend to meld over time.

Plan by taking a look at your schedule and setting aside particular periods for meal preparation. Having meals ready ahead of time lessens the temptation to choose easier, less nourishing options during hectic days.

In summary, implementing a thyroid-friendly meal plan necessitates giving careful thought to nutrient balance, meal prep techniques, and sample meal plans. People can proactively promote the health of their thyroid through nutrition by constructing well-balanced meals, creating meaningful sample meal plans, and utilizing effective meal prep procedures.

CHAPTER 5

BREAKFASTS THAT PROMOTE THYROID HEALTH

Bowls And Smoothies Packed With Nutrients

Adding nutrient-dense smoothies and bowls to your morning routine can have a revolutionary effect on thyroid health. These colorful mixtures serve as a nutritional powerhouse that specifically meets the needs of the thyroid gland.

Iodine, an essential mineral for thyroid function, is an important factor to take into account. You can assist thyroid hormone synthesis by including iodine-rich items in your smoothies, including seaweed or iodized salt.

Furthermore, these breakfast selections must contain antioxidants. Berries are an excellent source of antioxidants since they are high in vitamins C and E and can help fight oxidative stress and inflammation, two things that are frequently linked to thyroid issues. Leafy greens with high vitamin, mineral, and fiber content, such as kale or spinach, can improve the nutritional profile.

Including omega-3 fatty acids is also good when creating smoothie bowls that are healthy for the thyroid. Renowned for their omega-3 content, chia or flaxseeds not only add a creamy texture but also help thyroid health by balancing hormones and lowering inflammation.

These nutrient-dense breakfast options can be tailored to meet the needs and tastes of each individual.

To increase the amount of protein in your meal, promote satiety, and stabilize your blood sugar levels throughout the morning, try adding a scoop of Greek yogurt or protein powder that supports the thyroid.

<u>Whole Grain And High-Protein Choices</u>

Whole grain and high-protein breakfast alternatives are essential for thyroid health since they release energy and vital minerals gradually. Rich in fiber, whole grains such as quinoa, brown rice, and oats facilitate better digestion and blood sugar regulation. This is especially helpful for people who have thyroid abnormalities because stable blood sugar levels support good metabolic health in general.

Another essential component is protein, which helps to feel full and stimulates thyroid hormone synthesis. A balanced and thyroid-friendly diet can be promoted by including lean protein sources like eggs, lean meats, or plant-based options like tofu in your morning rotation.

In addition to satisfying hunger, combining whole grains with protein produces a potent nutritional synergy. For example, a quinoa and vegetable frittata combines the benefits of vibrant, nutrient-dense veggies with the availability of a full protein source. This combination of foods and flavors offers a range of vitamins and minerals that support thyroid function generally.

Those who choose breakfasts high in protein and whole grains can lay the groundwork for longer-lasting energy, enhanced metabolism, and better control of symptoms associated with their thyroid.

Simple and Fast Breakfast Recipes

Easy and quick breakfast recipes are quite helpful in this fast-paced world we live in, especially for thyroid-health-conscious people. These recipes encourage consistency in eating a thyroid-friendly diet by making sure that a healthy breakfast is available even on the busiest mornings.

The overnight oats phenomenon is one excellent fast breakfast alternative. Through the use of rolled oats and a preferred liquid (almond milk), as well as the addition of toppings (fruit, nuts, and seeds), people can make a heavy meal the night before. This not only saves time but also enables the liquid to be absorbed by the oats, giving them a delicious texture and a healthy start to the day.

A smoothie that is high in protein and vegetables is another quick and healthy breakfast option. Blending leafy greens, a source of protein, and fruits high in antioxidants results in a colorful cocktail that comes together quickly. This helps people prioritize their well-being because it not only improves thyroid health but also works with hectic schedules.

Convenience and nutrition go hand in hand, and quick and simple breakfast foods that support thyroid health are the perfect example of this. Through the adoption of these easily obtainable choices, people can effortlessly incorporate substances that promote thyroid function into their daily regimen, promoting a comprehensive approach to overall health.

CHAPTER 6

LUNCHES TO SUPPORT THE THYROID

Healthy Salads And Wraps For The Thyroid

Adding nutrient-dense salads and wraps to your lunchtime routine can make a huge difference in the area of thyroid health. These dishes are not only flavorful, but they also give the thyroid the nutrition it needs to perform at its best. Rich in vitamins A and K, dark leafy greens like kale and spinach—which are frequently included in these salads—also play important roles in maintaining thyroid function.

In particular, vitamin A is essential for the synthesis of thyroid hormones, and vitamin K promotes healthy calcium metabolism and aids in blood clotting.

Thyroid-boosting salads also frequently include items high in selenium, such as Brazil nuts, which is a necessary mineral for the conversion of thyroid hormones. By serving as a cofactor for the enzymes involved in this conversion process, selenium helps the body use thyroid hormones more effectively. The amino acids required for the production of thyroid hormones are provided by adding protein sources like quinoa or grilled chicken to these salads.

Wraps are also a thyroid-friendly option, particularly if you choose whole-grain wraps or low-carb lettuce leaves. Complex carbs included in whole grains like quinoa and brown rice provide steady blood sugar levels, which are essential for thyroid function since they release energy gradually. Additives high in omega-3, such as flaxseeds or salmon, wraps to intensify their thyroid-promoting qualities. Because of their well-known anti-inflammatory properties, omega-3 fatty acids may be helpful for those with autoimmune thyroid diseases like Hashimoto's thyroiditis.

Comforting and Filling Lunch Recipes

Not only can warm, filling lunch foods provide warmth, but they also provide a range of nutrients that help maintain thyroid function. It is especially vital to include meals high in iodine, which is essential for the manufacture of thyroid hormones. In recipes like warm grain bowls or fish-based soups, seafood—such as salmon and seaweed—is a great source of iodine. You can also carefully utilize iodized salt to make sure you're getting enough of this important mineral.

These recipes also frequently contain lean protein sources, such as chicken or turkey, which supply the amino acids required for the synthesis of thyroid hormones. Since zinc is essential in the control of thyroid function, foods high in zinc, such as lean meats and legumes, may also make their way into these warm meals. Including a selection of vibrant veggies also guarantees a varied spectrum of antioxidants, promoting general well-being and perhaps lowering inflammation, both of which can be advantageous for people with thyroid conditions.

Warm foods made with complex carbs, such as quinoa or sweet potatoes, provide you with long-lasting energy and help control your blood sugar. For those with thyroid abnormalities, stable blood sugar levels are essential since variations can affect hormone synthesis and worsen symptoms.

Options that are Office-Friendly and Portable

Lunch alternatives that are convenient to pack for the office and are portable help maintain thyroid health during hectic workdays. Making meals that are portable and quick to eat guarantees that people with thyroid issues can continue to follow their dietary requirements even when they have a busy schedule.

A thyroid-supportive bento box is a practical choice that offers several components that support thyroid health. This may include a section that contains lean protein—grilled chicken or tofu, for example—which supplies the amino acids required for the creation of thyroid hormones. A vibrant mix of veggies in another compartment can provide a variety of vitamins and minerals, such as vitamin A and selenium, which are essential for thyroid function.

To support thyroid function generally, include necessary fatty acids in a separate portion of the bento box with healthy fats like almonds or avocados. These fats assist the synthesis and use of thyroid hormones and are essential for hormone production and absorption.

Furthermore, adding a little portion of berries or other low-glycemic fruits to your diet offers antioxidants and a hint of sweetness without significantly raising your blood sugar levels.

Even on the busiest days, people can prioritize their thyroid health by preparing these portable and office-friendly thyroid-supportive alternatives, which will ensure a consistent supply of nutrients to promote normal thyroid function.

CHAPTER 7

DINNER RECIPES FORTHYROID FUNCTION

Thyroid-Friendly Protein Sources

Since protein is a necessary ingredient for good health in general, it becomes even more important for those who have thyroid problems to include thyroid-friendly protein sources in their supper meals. Lean protein choices aid in weight management, which is important for those with thyroid conditions.

Omega-3 fatty acids, which support thyroid function and have anti-inflammatory qualities, are found in salmon, making it a great option. Furthermore, lean poultry, such as turkey or chicken, is high in selenium, a mineral necessary for the metabolism of thyroid hormones.

Legumes are a great source of protein as well, especially lentils and chickpeas. The substantial fiber content of these plant-based proteins facilitates digestion and encourages a continuous release of energy. They also provide vital elements that are good for thyroid health, such as zinc and iron. For those looking for plant-based alternatives, quinoa, a complete protein, is a fantastic substitute. It is a great complement to a dinner that is thyroid-friendly because it contains all nine essential amino acids.

Another great approach to increasing protein consumption is to include eggs in dinner preparations. Iodine and selenium, which are both necessary for the synthesis of thyroid hormone, are abundant in eggs. Dinner ideas that use a range of these protein sources will guarantee a thyroid-supportive, well-rounded meal.

Dinner options for vegetarians and vegans

There is no shortage of nutrient-dense dinner options for those who are on a vegetarian or vegan diet to promote thyroid health. Since leafy greens are rich in vitamins, minerals, and antioxidants, they make great veggies, such as spinach and kale. These greens are part of a balanced diet that promotes thyroid health.

Tempeh and tofu are two essential plant-based proteins for vegetarian and vegan diets that are thyroid-friendly. Made from soybeans, tofu is a flexible ingredient that works well in a variety of recipes. It supports thyroid function overall by being an excellent supply of calcium, iron, and protein.

Another food made from soy, tempeh, is fermented to improve its digestibility and supply microorganisms that support gut health, which is associated with thyroid function.

A varied range of nutrients is ensured by adding a variety of bright vegetables to dinner meals, in addition to adding flavor and texture. Rich in vitamins and antioxidants, bell peppers, carrots, and sweet potatoes make for a well-rounded, thyroid-friendly dinner suitable for vegetarians or vegans.

Scrumptious and Packed with Nutrients Dinners

Making savory, nutrient-dense dinners is crucial to thyroid health maintenance. Spices and herbs add flavor to food and have several health advantages. For instance, the anti-inflammatory compound curcumin, which is found in turmeric, may help people with thyroid conditions.

Including healthy grains in dinner recipes, such as quinoa, brown rice, and oats, offers vital minerals and fiber. These grains support thyroid function in general and offer a consistent release of energy. Furthermore, high in fiber, antioxidants, and omega-3 fatty acids, nuts and seeds like chia and walnuts boost thyroid function.

Dinners can benefit from the flavor and nutritional benefits that fatty fish, such as sardines and mackerel, can bring. They contain high levels of omega-3 fatty acids, which support healthy thyroid function and have anti-inflammatory properties. People can make tasty, nutrient-dense dinners that support thyroid health by combining a range of bright vegetables, nutritious grains, and fragrant herbs and spices.

CHAPTER 8

SIDES AND SNACKS

Ideas For Thyroid-Healthy Snacks

Keeping the thyroid healthy is essential for general health, and eating the correct foods can help promote thyroid function. Snacking on nutrient-dense foods can give you the vital vitamins and minerals your thyroid needs.

A handful of mixed nuts, like Brazil nuts, walnuts, and almonds, is a great snack choice. Selenium, a trace mineral essential to thyroid function, is abundant in these nuts. As a potent antioxidant that shields the thyroid gland from oxidative damage, selenium is essential for the thyroid hormone conversion process.

Berries and Greek yogurt make another snack that's good for the thyroid. A great source of iodine, which is necessary for the generation of thyroid hormone, is Greek yogurt. Antioxidants from berries boost the body's defenses against inflammation and maintain a healthy thyroid.

Because seaweed contains a lot of iodine, it is also good for thyroid health. Since iodine is an essential part of thyroid hormones, adding seaweed to snacks can help satisfy the body's iodine needs. To prevent consuming too much iodine, it's crucial to eat seaweed in moderation.

Hummus and vegetable sticks combine to provide a filling and healthy snack. Chickpea-based hummus is high in protein and fiber, which helps with digestion and energy levels. Carrots and celery are among the veggies that provide extra vitamins and minerals that are essential for thyroid function.

Including these snacks in a well-balanced diet can help maintain normal thyroid function. However, to guarantee a wide range of nutrients that support general well-being, it's crucial to pay attention to portion sizes and keep a diversified diet.

High-Nutrient Side Dishes

Incorporating nutrient-dense side dishes that offer a diverse range of vitamins and minerals important for good thyroid function is crucial when focusing on thyroid health. These side dishes improve general well-being in addition to adding flavor to meals.

Quinoa salad with roasted veggies combines the health benefits of quinoa with vibrant vegetables in a side dish that is suitable for those with thyroid issues. While vegetables supply antioxidants and vital minerals like vitamins A and C, quinoa serves as a complete protein by providing all of the important amino acids. This combination encourages a well-rounded nutritional intake, which supports thyroid function.

A great source of beta-carotene, which is a precursor to vitamin A, is sweet potato wedges. Thyroid hormone synthesis depends on vitamin A, which also strengthens the immune system. Sweet potato wedges that have been roasted with a little olive oil added to boost beta-carotene absorption and give the dish a wonderful flavor.

An easy yet effective side dish for thyroid health is a sauté of leafy greens with garlic and olive oil. Leafy greens, such as kale and spinach, are high in magnesium, a mineral that is important for the synthesis and control of thyroid hormones. Additional antioxidants and anti-inflammatory qualities found in garlic help to maintain thyroid function overall.

A side dish high in protein and omega-3 fatty acids is salmon with lemon and herbs. These fats support a healthy inflammatory response in the body, which is essential for the function of the thyroid. Adding fatty fish, such as salmon, to side dishes gives you an extra nutritional boost that supports heart health and general well-being.

Everyday meals should include nutrient-dense side dishes so that people are getting all the nutrients they need for healthy thyroid function. To ensure that you are getting a wide range of vital nutrients, it's critical to keep your side dish options varied.

<u>Sugar-Free Sweets To Help Support The Thyroid</u>

Treating yourself doesn't have to harm your thyroid; in fact, including guilt-free snacks can be a fun way to promote thyroid function and sate your sweet tooth at the same time. It's important to select snacks that are high in nutrients that support the thyroid and low in processed sugars.

A trail mix made of nuts and dark chocolate is a tasty, guilt-free snack that combines the health benefits of almonds with the antioxidant-rich richness of dark chocolate. Flavonoids in dark chocolate help to maintain heart health, and antioxidants fight oxidative stress and improve thyroid function in general. Nuts that offer healthy fats and selenium, such as cashews and almonds, help to maintain optimal thyroid health.

Berries and chia seed pudding make a filling and healthy dessert choice. Chia seeds are high in fiber, protein, and omega-3 fatty acids. Additionally, these tiny seeds boost thyroid function by supplying vital minerals like phosphorus and magnesium. Berries give the treat an extra boost of antioxidants and a natural sweetness.

Energy balls made of coconut and almonds are a delightful and practical method to help thyroid function. Medium-chain triglycerides (MCTs), a good lipid that aids in energy metabolism, are found in coconuts. Vitamin E, magnesium, and selenium—all of which are essential for thyroid function—are found in almonds. When consumed in moderation, these nutrient-dense energy balls are a delightful treat.

A decadent and creamy dessert, avocado chocolate mousse also promotes thyroid health. Avocado supports thyroid function generally by being high in monounsaturated fats and a strong source of B vitamins and vitamin E. Rich chocolate taste is added without using too much sugar, and the antioxidant value is increased by the inclusion of dark cocoa powder.

In summary, including guilt-free snacks in a thyroid-friendly diet can enhance the pleasure of eating in general. Treats with nutritional value should be prioritized over refined sugars and processed components to maintain thyroid function in a well-rounded and supportive manner.

CHAPITRE 9

THYROID-EMPOWERED DRINKS

Herbal Infusions And Teas

Herbal infusions and teas are a great method to promote thyroid function naturally and gently keep things in balance. Some herbs are well known to have positive effects on the thyroid gland. Ashwagandha is one such plant. It is an adaptogen with a reputation for regulating the body's stress response, which has an indirect effect on thyroid function. Another plant that is frequently added to teas is ginseng, which can boost immunity and increase vitality in general.

Nettle tea is a noteworthy addition to recipes for thyroid health because of its abundant nutrient profile. Nettle is a rich source of minerals and vitamins, including iron, which is essential for those with thyroid conditions. Additionally, herbs like ginger and turmeric are great for supporting the thyroid because of their anti-inflammatory qualities. These components have the potential to lessen thyroid gland inflammation and support healthy thyroid function.

Herbs such as licorice root can also help to keep the adrenal glands healthy, which in turn helps the thyroid. When creating herbal teas, it's critical to maintain equilibrium to create a harmonic combination that supports various thyroid health issues. Including these teas in your daily routine might offer people who want to improve their thyroid function a consistent and healthy support system.

Drinks And Smoothies To Maintain Thyroid Balance

Smoothies have gained popularity as a practical and easy method to add thyroid-supporting foods to one's diet. Smoothies that are designed with the thyroid in mind can be nutrient-dense powerhouses that support thyroid hormone control. Antioxidant-rich fruits, like berries, are essential because they can fight against inflammation and oxidative stress, two main causes of thyroid dysfunction.

Because they are rich in vitamins and minerals, including iodine, leafy greens like spinach and kale are essential complements. Iodine is vital for thyroid health since it is a necessary nutrient for the synthesis of thyroid hormones. Furthermore, adding components high in omega-3s, such as flaxseeds and chia seeds, can help reduce inflammation overall and regulate thyroid hormones.

One noteworthy component that's frequently seen in smoothies that help the thyroid is coconut oil. Coconut oil's medium-chain fatty acids can improve metabolic performance, which may help those whose thyroid activity is slow. When these components are combined in a healthy ratio, the result is not only a tasty drink but also a nutritional boost that over time may have a good effect on thyroid function.

The Effect Of Hydration On Thyroid Function

Although it may not appear connected at first, staying hydrated is essential for thyroid function to be at its best. Sufficient water is essential for the thyroid gland to function properly and create hormones. Thyroid hormones need water to be transported throughout the body and to be converted from the inactive form, thyroxine, to the active form, triiodothyronine.

Thyroid hormone abnormalities can result from these mechanisms being disturbed by dehydration. Drinking too little water might cause the thyroid to produce fewer hormones, which could aggravate hypothyroidism symptoms. Furthermore, enough hydration helps the liver, which is an essential organ for the body's effective use of thyroid hormones by converting them.

Electrolytes are dissolved in water, including iodine and selenium, which are essential for thyroid function. The availability of these minerals may be compromised by dehydration, which could have a detrimental effect on thyroid function. To support the complex processes involved in thyroid hormone regulation and to guarantee optimal hydration, it is imperative to stress the drinking of clean, filtered water and herbal teas. Including hydration awareness in recipes for thyroid health emphasizes the multi-faceted approach required to keep the thyroid functioning properly.

CHAPTER 10

RECIPES FOR THYROID-HEALTHY OCCASIONS

Festive Recipes Using Thyroid-Friendly Substances

People who are concerned about their thyroid function can still enjoy delectable foods that support thyroid function on special occasions. Including foods that are beneficial to the thyroid in celebration meals helps to maintain general health and preserve the joy of the occasion.

Iodine, which is essential for the synthesis of thyroid hormones, is one component of thyroid health. Iodine-rich seafood, especially seaweed, makes for delicious additions to special menu items. Sushi with seaweed wraps, for example, is a great example of this. Furthermore, adding lean proteins like chicken or turkey can supply vital amino acids like tyrosine, which is a component of thyroid hormones.

Thyroid-supporting components, such as spinach, which is high in iron magnesium, and other vitamins and minerals, can improve celebratory salads. These minerals can enhance the color and nutritional density of a dish and are essential for thyroid function. Celebrate with salads and treats that include nuts and seeds, especially Brazil nuts and sunflower seeds, which are great providers of selenium, a mineral that supports thyroid function.

When it comes to desserts, choosing confections prepared with coconut flour rather than regular flour can be a thyroid-friendly decision. In addition to being gluten-free, coconut flour gives baked goods a delightful, nutty flavor. Incorporating antioxidant-rich berries can enhance thyroid health overall and add a delightful touch.

To put it simply, creating festive recipes with thyroid-friendly components is about choosing meals that promote thyroid function without sacrificing taste or appeal. People can enjoy special events while putting their thyroid health first by concentrating on iodine-rich foods, lean proteins, nutrient-dense veggies, and selenium-rich nuts and seeds.

Ideas For Festive And Holiday Meals

Food is a major component of celebrations and holidays, and people who have thyroid health issues can still enjoy these moments by selecting foods that are tasty and beneficial to thyroid function. Using nutrient-dense products and careful cooking techniques is key to creating thyroid-friendly holiday and celebratory meals.

A traditional Christmas main course, turkey is a great option for people who have thyroid issues. It is a lean protein source that also contains zinc and selenium, two important elements for thyroid function.

Herbs such as rosemary and thyme, when roasted with turkey, not only provide flavor but also antioxidants that are good for your health.

Festive meals require a side dish, and choices like sweet potatoes or roasted Brussels sprouts are not only tasty but also nutrient-dense and good for thyroid function. Rich in vitamins, minerals, and fiber, these veggies help maintain a thyroid-friendly diet that is well-balanced. Another inventive and wholesome substitute for classic bread stuffing is quinoa stuffing, which is produced with this grain that is high in protein.

Herbal teas, including chamomile or green tea, can be great options for beverages. During celebratory events, these teas provide hydration without the stimulating impacts of caffeinated options, encouraging a relaxed and thyroid-friendly ambiance.

Desserts may support thyroid health and still be decadent. Selecting dessert recipes that call for almond or coconut flour in place of refined flour offers a gluten-free and thyroid-friendly substitute. Dark chocolate, which is high in antioxidants, helps satiate sweet tooths and improve general health.

To summarize, nutrient-dense food selection, careful cooking methods, and inventive substitutions that balance taste and thyroid function are key components of holiday and celebratory meal ideas for those with thyroid issues.

Advice on Managing Social Events While Keeping Your Thyroid Health in Mind

For those whose thyroid health is a concern, attending social events can be difficult. However, with thoughtful preparation and understanding, these situations can be managed while placing a high priority on thyroid health. The following advice can help you have a thyroid-friendly time at social events:

1. **Communication is Key:** It may be important to let hosts or organizers know about any dietary limitations about thyroid health. This makes the social gathering more

pleasurable and stress-free by ensuring that solutions that suit individual needs are available.

2. Bring a Thyroid-Friendly meal: When it's suitable, bringing a meal that complies with thyroid-friendly recommendations guarantees that there will be a minimum of one choice that meets dietary needs. In addition to ensuring a safe decision, this proactive method enables the sharing of delectable, thyroid-healthy dishes with others.

3. Careful Menu Selections: People with thyroid issues should exercise caution when deciding what to choose from a menu at a social gathering or restaurant. Choosing whole grains, lean proteins, and vegetables that are high in nutrients will help create a meal that is well-balanced and promotes thyroid function.

4. It's Important to Stay Hydrated: Proper hydration is crucial for thyroid function. Selecting non-caffeinated beverages such as herbal teas or water during social gatherings aids in maintaining proper hydration levels without possibly interfering with thyroid function.

5. Moderation in Indulgences: Although delectable foods may be served during celebrations, moderation is key when it comes to enjoying them. The health of the thyroid may be adversely affected by eating diets high in processed components and refined sugars in excess. Enjoyment and health can coexist in harmony when you choose small servings and take time to fully appreciate the flavors.

6. Make sleep and stress management a priority. Social gatherings can occasionally cause sleep patterns to be disturbed and stress levels to rise. Getting enough sleep and managing stress are essential for thyroid health. Prioritizing sound sleep and implementing stress-relieving techniques like deep breathing or light exercise can improve general well-being both before and after social events.

In conclusion, proactive communication, careful menu selection, and a moderation approach to indulgence are all necessary for successfully navigating social occasions while keeping thyroid health in mind. People can maintain their thyroid health and enjoy social events by using these suggestions.

CHAPTER 11

FITNESS AND WAY OF LIFE FOR HEALTHY THYROID FUNCTION

Exercise's Significance For Thyroid Health

Engaging in physical activity is essential for general health and has a significant impact on thyroid function. Frequent exercise encourages the effective synthesis and conversion of thyroid hormones, which is essential for preserving thyroid health. Aerobic exercise increases the thyroid's ability to secrete hormones and stimulates the gland, as may jogging, cycling, or brisk walking.

Exercise also helps with weight management, which is important for thyroid health. It's crucial to keep a healthy weight to avoid diseases like hyperthyroidism and hypothyroidism. Thyroid dysfunction is frequently associated with obesity, and exercise helps reduce weight, which lowers the risk of thyroid-related problems.

An additional aspect of physical activity that can help thyroid health is resistance training. Strength training increases muscular mass, which can boost metabolism and increase the body's sensitivity to thyroid hormones. Consequently, this promotes general metabolic balance and aids in controlling thyroid function.

Striking a balance is essential, though, as too much activity can stress the body and perhaps interfere with thyroid function. As a result, people with thyroid disorders should customize their workout regimens to meet their unique demands and seek the guidance of medical professionals.

In conclusion, regular exercise is a powerful ally in preserving thyroid function. Exercise stimulates thyroid function in several ways, from helping to regulate weight to promoting hormone synthesis.

Techniques for Stress Management

There is a complex and significant relationship between thyroid health and stress. Long-term stress can negatively impact the thyroid gland, which can result in abnormalities in the synthesis and control of hormones. Stress triggers the body's "fight or flight" reaction, which results in the release of cortisol, a hormone that disrupts thyroid function when it is increased for long periods.

Using stress-reduction strategies that work is essential for people who want to maintain the health of their thyroid. It has been demonstrated that techniques like yoga, deep breathing, and meditation reduce tension and foster serenity. By limiting its prolonged increase and reducing its possible detrimental effects on the thyroid, these activities aid in the regulation of cortisol release.

In addition, having hobbies, going outside, and building strong social networks are essential elements of stress management. Developing a holistic approach to health can help to maintain a more balanced hormonal environment and reduce the negative effects of stress on the thyroid.

Stress management must be given top priority by those with thyroid disorders as part of their overall care strategy. Stress management practices can be positively correlated with thyroid function and long-term health by being incorporated into everyday living.

The Effects Of Sleep On Thyroid Function

It is impossible to overestimate the importance of getting enough healthy sleep for thyroid function as a cornerstone of overall health. The body goes through important processes that impact metabolism, hormone regulation, and overall physiological balance when we sleep. Sleep disturbances can have a significant effect on the thyroid gland.

Enough sleep, both restful and adequate, is necessary for thyroid hormone production and conversion to occur properly.

The body's internal clock, the circadian rhythm, is crucial in controlling thyroid function. Disturbances in this cycle, which are frequently brought on by inadequate sleep, can result in hormone imbalances, which in turn can aggravate thyroid disease.

In addition, lack of sleep can raise stress chemicals like cortisol, which is bad for thyroid function. Proper sleep hygiene should be prioritized because chronic sleep disturbances have been associated with a higher risk of thyroid diseases.

Supporting thyroid health requires establishing a regular sleep schedule, setting up a comfortable sleeping environment, and taking care of any underlying sleep issues.

People who have thyroid issues should prioritize getting enough sleep as part of their overall wellness plan because sleep and thyroid function are interdependent.

CHAPITRE 12

A 30-DAY DIET PLAN TO BOOST THYROID FUNCTION

The emphasis of the daily meal plan for increasing thyroid function is on including nutrient-dense meals that support thyroid function. here's a 30-day diet plan designed to support thyroid function:

Day 1

*Breakfast:

 Greek Yogurt With Berries And A Sprinkle Of Chia Seeds

- **Directions:** Simply mix a serving of Greek yogurt with a handful of fresh berries (such as strawberries, blueberries, or raspberries) and sprinkle with chia seeds for added fiber and omega-3 fatty acids.

*Snack:

Carrot Sticks With Hummus

- **Directions:** Wash and peel carrots, then slice into sticks. Serve with a side of hummus for dipping.

***Lunch:**

Grilled Chicken Salad With Spinach, Avocado, And Olive Oil Dressing

- **Directions:** Grill a seasoned chicken breast until fully cooked. Slice and serve over a bed of fresh spinach leaves, topped with sliced avocado. Drizzle with olive oil and a squeeze of lemon juice for dressing.

***Dinner:**

Baked Salmon With Steamed Broccoli And Quinoa

- **Directions:** Preheat your oven to 375°F (190°C). Place salmon fillets on a baking sheet lined with parchment paper. Season with salt, pepper, and your choice of herbs or spices. Bake for 12-15 minutes or until the salmon flakes easily with a fork. Steam broccoli until tender-crisp. Prepare quinoa according to package instructions. Serve salmon alongside steamed broccoli and quinoa.

Ensure to drink plenty of water throughout the day to stay hydrated. Enjoy your nutritious meals!

Day 2

***Breakfast:**

Scrambled Eggs With Spinach And Tomatoes.

- **Directions:** In a non-stick skillet, heat a small amount of olive oil over medium heat. Add chopped tomatoes and spinach leaves and sauté until wilted. In a bowl, whisk eggs and pour over the vegetables in the skillet. Stir gently until the eggs are cooked to your desired consistency. Season with salt and pepper to taste.

***Snack:**

Sliced Apple with Almond Butter.

- **Directions:** Wash and slice an apple into wedges. Spread almond butter on each apple slice for a satisfying and crunchy snack.

***Lunch:**

Lentil Soup.

- **Directions:** In a large pot, sauté diced onions, carrots, and celery in olive oil until softened. Add rinsed lentils, vegetable broth, diced tomatoes, and your choice of herbs and spices (such as thyme, oregano, and bay leaves). Bring to a boil, then reduce heat and simmer for about 20-25 minutes until the lentils are tender. Serve hot.

***Snack:**

Greek Yogurt with Cucumber Slices

- **Directions:** Slice a cucumber into thin rounds. Serve with a side of Greek yogurt for a refreshing and protein-packed snack.

***Dinner:**

Stir-Fried Tofu With Mixed Vegetables And Brown Rice

- **Directions:** Press tofu to remove excess moisture, then cut into cubes. In a wok or large skillet, heat olive oil over medium-high heat. Add tofu cubes and stir-fry until golden brown. Remove tofu from the skillet and set aside. In the same skillet, add more oil if needed and stir-fry mixed vegetables (such as bell peppers, broccoli, and snap peas) until tender-crisp. Add the tofu back to the skillet, along with soy sauce and your choice of seasonings. Serve over cooked brown rice.

<u>Day 3</u>

***Breakfast:**

Oatmeal topped with Sliced Bananas and a Drizzle of Honey

- **Directions:** Cook oats according to package instructions. Once cooked, top with sliced bananas and a drizzle of honey for natural sweetness.

***Snack:**

Cottage Cheese With Sliced Peaches.

- **Directions:** Scoop cottage cheese into a bowl and top with sliced peaches for a creamy and satisfying snack.

***Lunch:**

Turkey And Avocado Wrap With Whole Grain Tortilla

- **Directions:** Lay a whole grain tortilla flat. Spread mashed avocado over the tortilla, add sliced turkey breast, shredded lettuce, and any other desired fillings. Roll the tortilla tightly into a wrap and slice in half.

***Snack:**

Bell Pepper Strips with Guacamole

- **Directions:** Slice bell peppers into strips. Serve with a side of guacamole for a crunchy and flavorful snack.

***Dinner:**

Quinoa Salad with Roasted Vegetables and Feta Cheese

- **Directions:** Cook quinoa according to package instructions. Meanwhile, roast your favorite vegetables (such as bell peppers, zucchini, and cherry tomatoes) in the oven until tender. Combine cooked quinoa with roasted vegetables, crumbled feta cheese, chopped fresh herbs (such as parsley or basil), and a drizzle of olive oil and lemon juice for dressing.

<u>Day 4</u>

***Breakfast:**

Smoothie made with Spinach, Pineapple, Banana, and Coconut Milk

- **Directions:** In a blender, combine a handful of fresh spinach leaves, chunks of pineapple, a ripe banana, and coconut milk. Blend until smooth and creamy. Add more coconut milk if needed to reach your desired consistency.

***Snack:**

Trail Mix with Dried Fruit and Seeds

- **Directions:** Mix together your favorite combination of dried fruits (such as raisins, cranberries, or apricots), nuts (such as almonds, cashews, or walnuts), and seeds (such as pumpkin seeds or sunflower seeds) for a nutrient-packed snack.

***Lunch:**

Chickpea Salad

- **Directions:** In a bowl, combine cooked chickpeas, diced cucumber, cherry tomatoes, diced red onion, chopped fresh parsley, and crumbled feta cheese. Drizzle with olive oil and lemon juice, and season with salt and pepper to taste.

***Snack:**

Celery Sticks with Peanut Butter.

- **Directions:** Wash and cut celery stalks into sticks. Spread peanut butter on each celery stick for a crunchy and satisfying snack.

***Dinner:**

Grilled Shrimp Skewers with Roasted Sweet Potatoes and Asparagus

- **Directions:** Thread shrimp onto skewers and season with olive oil, garlic, lemon juice, and your choice of herbs (such as parsley or thyme). Grill until shrimp are pink and cooked through. Serve with roasted sweet potato chunks and asparagus spears tossed in olive oil, salt, and pepper, and roasted in the oven until tender.

<u>Day 5</u>

***Breakfast:**

Scrambled Tofu with Spinach and Tomatoes

- Directions: Crumble tofu in a skillet and sauté with chopped spinach and diced tomatoes until heated through. Season with turmeric, garlic powder, salt, and pepper for flavor.

***Snack:**

Sliced Pear with Almond Butter

- **Directions:** Slice a ripe pear and spread almond butter on each slice for a tasty and satisfying snack.

***Lunch:**

Quinoa and Black Bean Salad

- **Directions:** Combine cooked quinoa with black beans, diced bell peppers, corn kernels, chopped cilantro, and a squeeze of lime juice. Toss together and season with cumin, chili powder, salt, and pepper to taste.

***Snack:**

Greek Yogurt with Berries

- **Directions:** Spoon Greek yogurt into a bowl and top with fresh berries for a creamy and antioxidant-rich snack.

***Dinner:**

Baked Chicken Breast with Steamed Broccoli and Wild Rice

- **Directions:** Season chicken breasts with olive oil, garlic powder, paprika, salt, and pepper. Bake in the oven until cooked through. Serve with steamed broccoli florets and cooked wild rice.

Day 6

***Breakfast:**

Overnight Chia Seed Pudding with Berries

- **Directions:** In a jar, mix chia seeds with your choice of milk (such as almond milk or coconut milk) and a touch of honey or maple syrup. Stir well and refrigerate overnight. In the morning, top with fresh berries before serving.

***Snack:**

Handful of Walnuts with Dried Apricots

- **Directions:** Combine walnuts with dried apricots for a nutrient-rich and energizing snack.

***Lunch:**

Spinach and Feta Omelette

- **Directions:** Whisk eggs in a bowl and pour into a heated skillet. Add fresh spinach leaves and crumbled feta cheese to one half of the omelette. Once the eggs are cooked through, fold the omelette in half and serve.

***Snack:**

Carrot and Celery Sticks with Hummus.

- Directions: Wash and cut carrot and celery sticks. Serve with a side of hummus for dipping.

***Dinner:**

Turkey Meatballs with Zucchini Noodles.

- Directions: Mix ground turkey with breadcrumbs, minced garlic, chopped parsley, and an egg. Form into meatballs and bake in the oven until cooked through. Serve over spiralized zucchini noodles sautéed in olive oil and garlic.

Day 7

***Breakfast:**

Banana Walnut Oatmeal.

- **Directions:** Cook oats according to package instructions. Slice a banana and add it to the cooked oats along with chopped walnuts. Stir well and serve warm.

***Snack:**

Greek Yogurt with Honey and Almonds.

- **Directions:** Spoon Greek yogurt into a bowl and drizzle with honey. Sprinkle with sliced almonds for added crunch and flavor.

***Lunch:**

Grilled Veggie Wrap.

- Directions: Grill sliced vegetables such as zucchini, bell peppers, and onions until tender. Lay out a whole grain tortilla, spread hummus over it, and layer the grilled vegetables on top. Roll the tortilla tightly into a wrap and enjoy.

***Snack:**

Sliced Cucumber with Cottage Cheese.

- **Directions:** Slice a cucumber and serve with a side of cottage cheese for a refreshing and protein-packed snack.

***Dinner:**

Baked Salmon with Quinoa and Steamed Green Beans.

- **Directions:** Season salmon fillets with olive oil, lemon juice, and your choice of herbs (such as dill or parsley). Bake in the oven until cooked through. Serve with cooked quinoa and steamed green beans.

7!

Day 8

***Breakfast:**

Spinach and Mushroom Scramble.

- **Directions:** In a skillet, sauté sliced mushrooms until browned. Add a handful of fresh spinach leaves and cook until wilted. Pour beaten eggs over the vegetables and scramble until cooked through. Season with salt, pepper, and a sprinkle of grated cheese if desired.

***Snack:**

Apple Slices with Peanut Butter.

- Directions: Slice an apple and spread peanut butter on each slice for a satisfying and energizing snack.

***Lunch:**

Chicken Caesar Salad.

- **Directions:** Grill or bake chicken breast until cooked through. Slice and serve over a bed of romaine lettuce. Toss with Caesar dressing (homemade or store-bought) and top with grated Parmesan cheese and croutons.

***Snack:**

Greek Yogurt with Granola.

- **Directions:** Spoon Greek yogurt into a bowl and sprinkle with your favorite granola for a crunchy and protein-packed snack.

*Dinner:** Beef and Broccoli Stir-Fry with Brown Rice.

- **Directions:** Thinly slice beef steak and stir-fry in a hot skillet with sliced onions and minced garlic until browned. Add broccoli florets and stir-fry until tender-crisp. Pour in a mixture of soy sauce, ginger, and a touch of honey, and cook until heated through. Serve over cooked brown rice.

Day 9

*Breakfast:

Blueberry Almond Smoothie

- **Directions:** In a blender, combine almond milk, frozen blueberries, a ripe banana, a spoonful of almond butter, and a handful of spinach. Blend until smooth and creamy.

*Snack:

Trail Mix With Mixed Nuts And Dried Cranberries.

- **Directions:** Mix together mixed nuts (such as almonds, cashews, and walnuts) with dried cranberries for a portable and nutritious snack.

***Lunch:**

Turkey and Avocado Wrap.

- **Directions:** Lay out a whole grain tortilla and spread mashed avocado over it. Layer sliced turkey breast, lettuce, tomato, and cucumber on top. Roll tightly into a wrap and slice in half.

***Snack:**

Carrot Sticks with Hummus.

- **Directions:** Wash and peel carrots, then slice into sticks. Serve with a side of hummus for dipping.

***Dinner:**

Lemon Garlic Shrimp With Quinoa And Steamed Asparagus.

- **Directions:** Marinate shrimp in a mixture of lemon juice, minced garlic, olive oil, and Italian herbs for about 30 minutes. Sauté the shrimp in a skillet until pink and cooked through. Serve over cooked quinoa and steamed asparagus.

Day 10

*Breakfast:

Greek Yogurt Parfait with Berries and Granola.

- **Directions:** In a glass or bowl, layer Greek yogurt with fresh berries (such as strawberries, blueberries, or raspberries) and granola. Repeat layers as desired.

**Snack:

Handful of Mixed Berries (e.g., strawberries, blueberries, raspberries).

- **Directions:** Simply wash the berries and enjoy them as a refreshing and nutritious snack.

*Lunch:

Spinach and Chickpea Salad with Lemon Tahini Dressing.

- **Directions:** Toss together fresh spinach leaves, cooked chickpeas, sliced cucumber, cherry tomatoes, and crumbled feta cheese. Drizzle with a mixture of tahini, lemon juice, garlic, and a splash of water to thin.

***Snack:**

Celery Sticks with Almond Butter.

- **Directions:** Wash and cut celery stalks into sticks. Spread almond butter on each celery stick for a crunchy and satisfying snack.

***Dinner:**

Grilled Chicken with Roasted Sweet Potatoes and Steamed Broccoli

- **Directions:** Marinate chicken breasts in a mixture of olive oil, lemon juice, minced garlic, and your choice of herbs (such as thyme or rosemary). Grill until cooked through. Serve with roasted sweet potato wedges tossed in olive oil, paprika, and salt, alongside steamed broccoli.

Day 11

***Breakfast:**

Veggie Omelette with Feta Cheese.

- **Directions:** In a non-stick skillet, sauté diced bell peppers, onions, and spinach until softened. Pour beaten eggs over the vegetables and cook until set. Crumble feta cheese over one half of the omelette and fold it in half. Cook for another minute until the cheese melts.

***Snack:**

Sliced Mango with Cottage Cheese

- **Directions:** Peel and slice a ripe mango. Serve with a side of cottage cheese for a creamy and sweet snack.

***Lunch:**

Quinoa Salad with Roasted Vegetables and Balsamic Vinaigrette

- **Directions:** Cook quinoa according to package instructions. Roast diced vegetables (such as bell peppers, zucchini, and eggplant) in the oven until tender. Toss the cooked quinoa with the roasted vegetables and drizzle with balsamic vinaigrette.

***Snack:**

Greek Yogurt with Almonds and Honey.

- Directions: Spoon Greek yogurt into a bowl and top with sliced almonds and a drizzle of honey for a protein-rich and satisfying snack.

***Dinner:**

Baked Cod with Lemon and Herbs, Served with Steamed Green Beans

- **Directions:** Place cod fillets on a baking sheet lined with parchment paper. Drizzle with olive oil and lemon juice, and sprinkle with chopped fresh herbs (such as parsley or dill), salt, and pepper. Bake in the oven until the fish is opaque and flakes easily with a fork. Serve with steamed green beans on the side.

Day 12

***Breakfast:**

Berry Spinach Smoothie

- **Directions:** In a blender, combine a handful of spinach, frozen mixed berries (such as strawberries, blueberries, and raspberries), a banana, Greek yogurt, and a splash of almond milk. Blend until smooth and creamy.

***Snack:**

Handful of Walnuts with Dried Apricots.

- **Directions:** Combine walnuts with dried apricots for a satisfying and nutritious snack.

*Lunch:

 Turkey and Hummus Wrap with Mixed Greens

- **Directions:** Spread hummus on a whole grain wrap, layer with sliced turkey breast, mixed greens, cucumber slices, and shredded carrots. Roll tightly and slice in half.

*Snack:

Carrot Sticks with Guacamole.

- **Directions:** Wash and peel carrots, then slice into sticks. Serve with a side of guacamole for dipping.

*Dinner:

 Lentil and Vegetable Soup.

- **Directions:** In a large pot, sauté diced onions, carrots, and celery in olive oil until softened. Add rinsed lentils, diced tomatoes, vegetable broth, and your choice of vegetables (such as spinach, kale, or zucchini). Season with herbs and spices (such as cumin, paprika, and thyme). Simmer until the lentils and vegetables are tender. Serve hot.

<u>Day 13</u>

***Breakfast:**

Greek Yogurt Bowl with Chopped Nuts and Honey.

- **Directions:** Scoop Greek yogurt into a bowl. Top with chopped nuts (such as almonds, walnuts, or pecans) and a drizzle of honey for sweetness.

***Snack:**

Sliced Apple with Almond Butter.

- **Directions:** Slice an apple and spread almond butter on each slice for a satisfying and crunchy snack.

***Lunch:**

Spinach And Quinoa Stuffed Bell Peppers.

- **Directions:** Cook quinoa according to package instructions. In a bowl, mix cooked quinoa with sautéed spinach, diced tomatoes, black beans, and shredded cheese. Stuff the mixture into halved bell peppers, place them in a baking dish, and bake until the peppers are tender and the filling is heated through.

***Snack:**

Cottage Cheese with Pineapple Chunks.

- **Directions:** Spoon cottage cheese into a bowl and top with chunks of fresh pineapple for a refreshing and protein-rich snack.

***Dinner:**

Baked Chicken Thighs with Roasted Brussels Sprouts and Sweet Potatoes

- **Directions:** Season chicken thighs with olive oil, garlic powder, paprika, salt, and pepper. Bake in the oven until cooked through. Serve with roasted Brussels sprouts and cubed sweet potatoes tossed in olive oil, salt, and pepper.

Day 14

***Breakfast:**

Avocado Toast with Poached Eggs.

- Directions: Toast whole grain bread slices. Mash ripe avocado onto the toast and top with poached eggs. Season with salt, pepper, and a sprinkle of red pepper flakes if desired.

***Snack:**

Mixed Berry Smoothie.

- **Directions:** Blend together a mixture of mixed berries (such as strawberries, blueberries, and raspberries) with Greek yogurt, a banana, and a splash of almond milk until smooth.

***Lunch:**

Tuna Salad Lettuce Wraps

- **Directions:** Mix canned tuna with diced celery, red onion, and mayonnaise. Spoon the tuna salad onto large lettuce leaves and roll them up to create wraps.

***Snack:**

Carrot and Celery Sticks with Hummus.

- **Directions:** Wash and cut carrot and celery sticks. Serve with a side of hummus for dipping.

***Dinner:**

Grilled Salmon with Roasted Asparagus and Quinoa.

- **Directions:** Season salmon fillets with olive oil, lemon juice, garlic, and dill. Grill until cooked through. Serve with roasted asparagus spears and cooked quinoa.

Day 15

***Breakfast:**

Banana Nut Overnight Oats.

- **Directions:** In a jar or container, mix rolled oats with mashed banana, chopped nuts (such as walnuts or almonds), a dash of cinnamon, and your choice of milk (such as almond milk or oat milk). Stir well, cover, and refrigerate overnight. Enjoy cold in the morning.

***Snack:**

Handful of Mixed Nuts and Dried Cranberries.

- **Directions:** Combine mixed nuts (such as almonds, cashews, and pistachios) with dried cranberries for a nutritious and energizing snack.

***Lunch:**

Chicken and Quinoa Salad.

- **Directions:** Cook quinoa according to package instructions. In a bowl, combine cooked quinoa with diced grilled chicken breast, cherry tomatoes, cucumber slices, avocado cubes, and crumbled feta cheese. Drizzle with balsamic vinaigrette and toss to coat.

***Snack:**

Greek Yogurt with Berries and Honey.

- **Directions:** Spoon Greek yogurt into a bowl and top with fresh berries (such as strawberries, blueberries, or raspberries). Drizzle with honey for sweetness.

***Dinner:**

Turkey Meatball Pasta with Spinach.

- Directions: Cook whole grain pasta according to package instructions. Meanwhile, bake turkey meatballs in the oven until cooked through. In a skillet, sauté minced garlic in olive oil until fragrant, then add fresh spinach and cook until wilted. Toss cooked pasta with marinara sauce, spinach, and turkey meatballs. Serve hot.

Day 16

***Breakfast:**

Veggie and Cheese Breakfast Quesadilla.

- **Directions:** Heat a whole grain tortilla in a skillet. Sprinkle shredded cheese (such as cheddar or mozzarella) on one half of the tortilla. Top with sautéed vegetables (such as bell peppers, onions, and mushrooms). Fold the tortilla in half and cook until the cheese is melted and the tortilla is golden brown on both sides.

***Snack:**

Apple Slices with Peanut Butter

- **Directions:** Slice an apple and spread peanut butter on each slice for a satisfying and energizing snack.

***Lunch:**

Mediterranean Chickpea Salad

- **Directions:** In a bowl, combine cooked chickpeas, diced cucumber, cherry tomatoes, chopped red onion, Kalamata olives, and crumbled feta cheese. Drizzle with olive oil, lemon juice, and a sprinkle of dried oregano. Toss to combine.

***Snack:**

Cottage Cheese with Pineapple Chunks.

- **Directions:** Spoon cottage cheese into a bowl and top with chunks of fresh pineapple for a refreshing and protein-rich snack.

***Dinner:**

Baked Cod with Lemon and Herbs, Served with Quinoa and Steamed Broccoli

- **Directions:** Place cod fillets on a baking sheet lined with parchment paper. Drizzle with olive oil, lemon juice, minced garlic, and chopped fresh herbs (such as parsley or dill). Bake in the oven until the fish is opaque and flakes easily with a fork. Serve with cooked quinoa and steamed broccoli.

Day 17

***Breakfast:**

Berry Spinach Smoothie Bowl.

- **Directions:** In a blender, combine spinach, mixed berries (such as strawberries, blueberries, and raspberries), banana, Greek yogurt, and a splash of almond milk. Blend until smooth and pour into a bowl. Top with granola, sliced almonds, and additional berries.

***Snack:**

Handful of Trail Mix with Dried Fruit and Nuts

- **Directions:** Mix together your favorite combination of dried fruits (such as raisins, cranberries, or apricots) and nuts (such as almonds, cashews, or walnuts) for a portable and energizing snack.

***Lunch:**

Grilled Chicken Caesar Salad.

- **Directions:** Grill chicken breast until fully cooked. Slice and serve over a bed of romaine lettuce. Drizzle with Caesar dressing and sprinkle with grated Parmesan cheese and croutons.

***Snack:**

Sliced Cucumber with Hummus.

- **Directions:** Wash and slice a cucumber. Serve with a side of hummus for a refreshing and satisfying snack.

***Dinner:**

Turkey and Vegetable Stir-Fry with Brown Rice.

- **Directions:** In a wok or large skillet, stir-fry sliced turkey breast with mixed vegetables (such as bell peppers, broccoli, and snap peas) in a mixture of soy sauce, garlic, and ginger. Serve over cooked brown rice.

Day 18

***Breakfast:**

Avocado Toast with Poached Eggs.

- **Directions:** Toast whole grain bread slices. Mash ripe avocado onto the toast and top with poached eggs. Season with salt, pepper, and a sprinkle of red pepper flakes if desired.

***Snack:**

Greek Yogurt with Mixed Berries.

- **Directions:** Spoon Greek yogurt into a bowl and top with mixed berries (such as strawberries, blueberries, and raspberries) for a creamy and antioxidant-rich snack.

***Lunch:**

Quinoa and Black Bean Stuffed Bell Peppers.

- **Directions:** Cook quinoa according to package instructions. In a bowl, mix cooked quinoa with black beans, diced tomatoes, corn kernels, chopped cilantro, and a squeeze of lime juice. Stuff the mixture into halved bell peppers and bake until peppers are tender.

***Snack:**

Carrot Sticks with Hummus.

- **Directions:** Wash and cut carrot sticks. Serve with a side of hummus for a crunchy and satisfying snack.

***Dinner:**

Baked Salmon with Roasted Asparagus and Sweet Potatoes.

- **Directions:** Season salmon fillets with olive oil, lemon juice, minced garlic, and your choice of herbs (such as dill or parsley). Bake in the oven until cooked through. Serve with roasted asparagus spears and sweet potato wedges roasted until tender.

Day 19

***Breakfast:**

Spinach and Feta Breakfast Wrap.

- **Directions:** In a skillet, sauté fresh spinach until wilted. In a whole grain tortilla, add scrambled eggs, sautéed spinach, and crumbled feta cheese. Roll up the tortilla and enjoy.

***Snack:**

Apple Slices with Almond Butter.

- **Directions:** Slice an apple and spread almond butter on each slice for a satisfying and energizing snack.

***Lunch:**

Mediterranean Chickpea Salad.

- **Directions:** Combine cooked chickpeas, diced cucumber, cherry tomatoes, chopped red onion, Kalamata olives, and crumbled feta cheese in a bowl. Drizzle with olive oil, lemon juice, and sprinkle with dried oregano. Toss gently to combine.

***Snack:**

Greek Yogurt with Honey and Walnuts.

- **Directions:** Spoon Greek yogurt into a bowl, drizzle with honey, and sprinkle with chopped walnuts for added crunch and flavor.

***Dinner:**

Turkey Meatball Pasta with Zucchini Noodles.

- **Directions:** Bake turkey meatballs in the oven until cooked through. Spiralize zucchini into noodles and sauté in a skillet with olive oil and garlic until tender. Toss with marinara sauce and serve with turkey meatballs on top.

<u>**Day 20**</u>

***Breakfast:**

Banana Almond Smoothie.

- **Directions:** Blend together a ripe banana, almond milk, a scoop of almond butter, and a handful of spinach until smooth and creamy.

***Snack:**

Trail Mix with Mixed Nuts and Dried Fruit.

- **Directions:** Combine mixed nuts (such as almonds, cashews, and walnuts) with dried fruit (such as raisins, cranberries, and apricots) for a nutritious and energizing snack.

***Lunch:**

Greek Salad with Grilled Chicken.

- **Directions**: Toss together chopped romaine lettuce, sliced cucumber, cherry tomatoes, Kalamata olives, red onion, and feta cheese. Top with grilled chicken breast and drizzle with olive oil and red wine vinegar.

***Snack:**

Sliced Cucumber with Hummus.

- **Directions:** Wash and slice a cucumber. Serve with a side of hummus for a crunchy and refreshing snack.

***Dinner:**

Baked Cod with Lemon and Herbs, Served with Quinoa and Steamed Broccoli

- **Directions:** Season cod fillets with olive oil, lemon juice, minced garlic, and chopped fresh herbs (such as parsley or dill). Bake in the oven until the fish is opaque and flakes easily with a fork. Serve with cooked quinoa and steamed broccoli.

Day 21

***Breakfast:**

Scrambled Tofu with Spinach and Tomatoes.

- **Directions:** Crumble tofu in a skillet and sauté with chopped spinach and diced tomatoes until heated through.

Season with turmeric, garlic powder, salt, and pepper for flavor.

***Snack:**

Mixed Berry Smoothie

- **Directions:** Blend together mixed berries (such as strawberries, blueberries, and raspberries), Greek yogurt, a banana, and a splash of almond milk until smooth and creamy.

***Lunch:**

Lentil and Vegetable Soup.

- **Directions:** In a large pot, sauté diced onions, carrots, and celery in olive oil until softened. Add rinsed lentils, diced tomatoes, vegetable broth, and your choice of vegetables (such as spinach, kale, or zucchini). Season with herbs and spices (such as cumin, paprika, and thyme). Simmer until the lentils and vegetables are tender. Serve hot.

***Snack:**

Carrot Sticks with Hummus.

- **Directions:** Wash and peel carrots, then slice into sticks. Serve with a side of hummus for dipping.

***Dinner:**

Grilled Salmon with Roasted Sweet Potatoes and Asparagus

- **Directions:** Season salmon fillets with olive oil, lemon juice, minced garlic, and your choice of herbs. Grill until cooked through. Serve with roasted sweet potato wedges and asparagus spears roasted until tender.

Day 22

Breakfast:* Berry Spinach Smoothie Bowl.

- **Directions:** Blend together spinach, mixed berries (such as strawberries, blueberries, and raspberries), banana, Greek yogurt, and a splash of almond milk until smooth. Pour into a bowl and top with granola, sliced almonds, and additional berries.

***Snack:**

Greek Yogurt with Honey and Almonds.

- **Directions**: Spoon Greek yogurt into a bowl, drizzle with honey, and sprinkle with chopped almonds for added crunch and flavor.

***Lunch:**

Quinoa Salad with Grilled Vegetables.

- **Directions:** Cook quinoa according to package instructions. Grill mixed vegetables (such as bell peppers, zucchini, and eggplant) until tender. Toss the grilled vegetables with cooked quinoa, chopped fresh herbs (such as parsley or basil), and a squeeze of lemon juice. Season with salt and pepper to taste.

***Snack:**

Sliced Apple with Peanut Butter.

- **Directions:** Slice an apple and spread peanut butter on each slice for a satisfying and nutritious snack.

***Dinner:**

Turkey and Black Bean Lettuce Wraps.

- **Directions:** In a skillet, cook ground turkey with diced onion, minced garlic, and taco seasoning until browned. Add black beans and cook until heated through. Spoon the turkey mixture onto large lettuce leaves, top with diced tomatoes, avocado slices, and a dollop of Greek yogurt.

Day 23

***Breakfast:**

Greek Yogurt Parfait with Berries and Granola.

- **Directions:** Layer Greek yogurt with fresh berries (such as strawberries, blueberries, or raspberries) and granola in a glass or bowl. Repeat layers as desired.

***Snack:**

Handful of Trail Mix with Nuts and Dried Fruit.

- **Directions:** Combine mixed nuts (such as almonds, cashews, and walnuts) with dried fruit (such as raisins, cranberries, and apricots) for a portable and energizing snack.

***Lunch:**

Chickpea and Avocado Salad.

- **Directions:** In a bowl, combine chickpeas, diced avocado, cherry tomatoes, cucumber slices, red onion, and fresh cilantro. Drizzle with olive oil and lemon juice, and season with salt and pepper to taste.

*Snack:

 Carrot Sticks with Hummus.

- **Directions:** Wash and cut carrot sticks. Serve with a side of hummus for a crunchy and satisfying snack.

Dinner: Baked Chicken Breast with Quinoa and Steamed Broccoli.

- **Directions:** Season chicken breast with olive oil, garlic powder, paprika, salt, and pepper. Bake in the oven until cooked through. Serve with cooked quinoa and steamed broccoli on the side.

Day 24

***Breakfast:**

Scrambled Eggs with Spinach and Tomatoes.

- **Directions:** In a skillet, sauté spinach and diced tomatoes until wilted. Pour beaten eggs over the vegetables and scramble until cooked through. Season with salt, pepper, and a sprinkle of grated cheese if desired.

***Snack:**

Greek Yogurt with Mixed Berries.

- **Directions:** Spoon Greek yogurt into a bowl and top with mixed berries (such as strawberries, blueberries, and raspberries) for a creamy and antioxidant-rich snack.

***Lunch:**

Turkey and Hummus Wrap with Whole Grain Tortilla.

- **Directions:** Spread hummus on a whole grain tortilla. Add sliced turkey breast, lettuce, cucumber, and tomato. Roll up the tortilla and slice in half.

***Snack:**

Sliced Cucumber with Cottage Cheese

- **Directions:** Wash and slice a cucumber. Serve with a side of cottage cheese for a refreshing and protein-packed snack.

***Dinner:**

Grilled Salmon with Roasted Vegetables

- **Directions:** Season salmon fillets with olive oil, lemon juice, minced garlic, and your choice of herbs. Grill until cooked through. Serve with roasted mixed vegetables (such as bell peppers, zucchini, and carrots) seasoned with olive oil, salt, and pepper.

Day 25

***Breakfast:**

Banana Nut Oatmeal.

- **Directions:** Cook oats according to package instructions. Slice a banana and add it to the cooked oats along with a sprinkle of chopped nuts (such as walnuts or almonds) and a drizzle of honey or maple syrup for sweetness.

***Snack:**

Handful of Mixed Berries (e.g., strawberries, blueberries, raspberries).

- **Directions:** Wash the berries and enjoy them as a refreshing and nutritious snack.

***Lunch:**

Quinoa and Black Bean Salad

- Directions: Combine cooked quinoa with black beans, diced bell peppers, corn kernels, chopped cilantro, and a squeeze of lime juice. Toss together and season with cumin, chili powder, salt, and pepper to taste.

***Snack:**

Carrot Sticks with Hummus.

- **Directions:** Wash and peel carrots, then slice into sticks. Serve with a side of hummus for a crunchy and satisfying snack.

***Dinner:**

Baked Chicken Thighs with Roasted Brussels Sprouts and Sweet Potatoes

- **Directions:** Season chicken thighs with olive oil, garlic powder, paprika, salt, and pepper. Bake in the oven until cooked through. Serve with roasted Brussels sprouts and cubed sweet potatoes tossed in olive oil, salt, and pepper.

Day 26

*Breakfast:

Veggie and Cheese Breakfast Quesadilla.

- **Directions:** Heat a whole grain tortilla in a skillet. Sprinkle shredded cheese (such as cheddar or mozzarella) on one half of the tortilla. Top with sautéed vegetables (such as bell peppers, onions, and mushrooms). Fold the tortilla in half and cook until the cheese is melted and the tortilla is golden brown on both sides.

*Snack:

Greek Yogurt with Berries and Honey.

- **Directions:** Spoon Greek yogurt into a bowl, top with fresh berries (such as strawberries, blueberries, or raspberries), and drizzle with honey for sweetness.

***Lunch:**

Mediterranean Chickpea Salad.

- **Directions:** Combine cooked chickpeas, diced cucumber, cherry tomatoes, chopped red onion, Kalamata olives, and crumbled feta cheese in a bowl. Drizzle with olive oil, lemon juice, and sprinkle with dried oregano. Toss gently to combine.

***Snack:**

Sliced Apple with Almond Butter.

- **Directions:** Slice an apple and spread almond butter on each slice for a satisfying and nutritious snack.

***Dinner:**

Grilled Salmon with Quinoa and Steamed Broccoli

- **Directions:** Season salmon fillets with olive oil, lemon juice, minced garlic, and your choice of herbs. Grill until cooked through. Serve with cooked quinoa and steamed broccoli on the side.

<u>**Day 27**</u>

***Breakfast:**

Spinach and Feta Omelette.

- **Directions:** Whisk eggs in a bowl and pour into a heated skillet. Add fresh spinach leaves and crumbled feta cheese to one half of the omelette. Once the eggs are cooked through, fold the omelette in half and serve.

***Snack:**

Sliced Pear with Almond Butter.

- **Directions:** Slice a ripe pear and spread almond butter on each slice for a tasty and satisfying snack.

***Lunch:**

Turkey and Avocado Wrap

- **Directions:** Lay out a whole grain tortilla and spread mashed avocado over it. Layer sliced turkey breast, lettuce, tomato, and cucumber on top. Roll tightly into a wrap and slice in half.

***Snack:**

Carrot Sticks with Hummus.

- **Directions:** Wash and cut carrot and celery sticks. Serve with a side of hummus for dipping.

***Dinner:**

Baked Cod with Lemon and Herbs, Served with Roasted Vegetables

- **Directions:** Season cod fillets with olive oil, lemon juice, minced garlic, and chopped fresh herbs (such as parsley or dill). Bake in the oven until the fish is opaque and flakes easily with a fork. Serve with roasted mixed vegetables (such as bell peppers, zucchini, and carrots) seasoned with olive oil, salt, and pepper.

Day 28

***Breakfast:**

Greek Yogurt Parfait with Berries and Granola.

- **Directions:** Layer Greek yogurt with fresh berries (such as strawberries, blueberries, or raspberries) and granola in a glass or bowl. Repeat layers as desired.

***Snack:**

Handful of Trail Mix with Nuts and Dried Fruit.

- **Directions:** Combine mixed nuts (such as almonds, cashews, and walnuts) with dried fruit (such as raisins, cranberries, and apricots) for a portable and energizing snack.

***Lunch:**

Chicken Caesar Salad

- **Directions:** Grill or bake chicken breast until cooked through. Slice and serve over a bed of romaine lettuce. Drizzle with Caesar dressing and sprinkle with grated Parmesan cheese and croutons.

***Snack:**

Sliced Cucumber with Hummus.

- **Directions:** Wash and slice a cucumber. Serve with a side of hummus for a crunchy and refreshing snack.

***Dinner:**

Lentil and Vegetable Soup.

- **Directions:** In a large pot, sauté diced onions, carrots, and celery in olive oil until softened. Add rinsed lentils, diced tomatoes, vegetable broth, and your choice of vegetables (such as spinach, kale, or zucchini). Season with herbs and spices (such as cumin, paprika, and thyme). Simmer until the lentils and vegetables are tender. Serve hot.

Day 29

***Breakfast:**

Banana Walnut Oatmeal

- **Directions:** Cook oats according to package instructions. Slice a banana and add it to the cooked oats along with chopped walnuts. Stir well and serve warm.

***Snack:**

Greek Yogurt with Honey and Almonds.

- **Directions:** Spoon Greek yogurt into a bowl and drizzle with honey. Sprinkle with sliced almonds for added crunch and flavor.

***Lunch:**

Grilled Chicken Salad with Avocado and Olive Oil Dressing

- **Directions:** Grill chicken breast until cooked through. Slice and serve over a bed of mixed greens. Top with sliced avocado and drizzle with olive oil and balsamic vinegar.

***Snack:**

Carrot Sticks with Hummus

- **Directions:** Wash and cut carrot sticks. Serve with a side of hummus for a crunchy and satisfying snack.

***Dinner:**

Baked Salmon with Quinoa and Steamed Broccoli

- **Directions:** Season salmon fillets with olive oil, lemon juice, minced garlic, and your choice of herbs (such as dill or parsley). Bake in the oven until cooked through. Serve with cooked quinoa and steamed broccoli.

Day 30

*Breakfast:

Spinach and Mushroom Scramble.

- **Directions:** In a skillet, sauté sliced mushrooms until browned. Add a handful of fresh spinach leaves and cook until wilted. Pour beaten eggs over the vegetables and scramble until cooked through. Season with salt, pepper, and a sprinkle of grated cheese if desired.

*Snack:

Mixed Berry Smoothie

- **Directions:** Blend together mixed berries (such as strawberries, blueberries, and raspberries), Greek yogurt, a banana, and a splash of almond milk until smooth and creamy.

*Lunch:

Turkey and Avocado Wrap.

- **Directions:** Lay out a whole grain tortilla and spread mashed avocado over it. Layer sliced turkey breast, lettuce, tomato, and cucumber on top. Roll tightly into a wrap and slice in half.

***Snack:**

Greek Yogurt with Berries and Honey.

- Directions: Spoon Greek yogurt into a bowl and top with fresh berries (such as strawberries, blueberries, or raspberries). Drizzle with honey for sweetness.

***Dinner:**

Grilled Chicken with Roasted Vegetables

- Directions: Marinate chicken breasts in a mixture of olive oil, lemon juice, minced garlic, and your choice of herbs. Grill until cooked through. Serve with roasted mixed vegetables (such as bell peppers, zucchini, and carrots) seasoned with olive oil, salt, and pepper.

Throughout the month, ensure you stay hydrated by drinking plenty of water and herbal teas. Limit processed foods, refined sugars, and excessive caffeine intake, as these can negatively impact thyroid function. Additionally, consider incorporating iodine-rich foods like seaweed, selenium-rich foods like Brazil nuts, and zinc-rich foods like pumpkin seeds into your meals for added thyroid support. Always consult with a healthcare professional before making significant dietary changes, especially if you have thyroid issues or are on medication.

Shopping Lists And Advice On Getting Ready

Embarking on a journey towards thyroid wellness is both empowering and transformative. As you navigate the aisles of the grocery store, your choices become the building blocks of your vitality. Here, I offer you a comprehensive shopping list and invaluable advice to support your thyroid diet journey:

<u>Fresh Produce</u>

1. Leafy Greens: Spinach, kale, Swiss chard - rich in vitamins and minerals crucial for thyroid health.

2. Colorful Vegetables: Carrots, bell peppers, and sweet potatoes - packed with antioxidants and beta-carotene to support thyroid function.

3. Cruciferous Vegetables: Broccoli, cauliflower, Brussels sprouts - while these are often advised to be consumed in moderation due to their goitrogenic properties, cooking them lightly can mitigate their impact.

4. Berries: Blueberries, strawberries, raspberries - excellent sources of antioxidants and fiber to combat inflammation.

5. Citrus Fruits: Oranges, lemons, grapefruits - high in vitamin C, which aids in the absorption of iron and supports immune function.

Protein Sources

6. Lean Meats: Skinless chicken breast, turkey, lean cuts of beef - rich in protein and zinc, essential for thyroid hormone production.

7. Fatty Fish: Salmon, trout, mackerel - abundant in omega-3 fatty acids, which reduce inflammation and support thyroid function.

8. Legumes: Lentils, chickpeas, black beans - great plant-based sources of protein, fiber, and essential nutrients.

9. Eggs: A complete protein source, containing selenium and iodine, vital for thyroid health.

10. Nuts and Seeds: Brazil nuts, pumpkin seeds, almonds - rich in selenium and other micronutrients crucial for thyroid function.

Whole Grains and Healthy Fats

11. Whole Grains: Quinoa, brown rice, oats - provide complex carbohydrates and fiber for sustained energy levels.

12. Healthy Fats: Avocado, olive oil, flaxseed oil – essential for hormone production and overall cellular health.

Dairy and Alternatives

13. Greek Yogurt: High in protein and probiotics, beneficial for gut health.

14. Almond Milk: A dairy-free alternative fortified with calcium and vitamin D.

15. Cheese: Opt for low-fat varieties like feta or mozzarella, in moderation.

Herbs, Spices, And Condiments

16. Turmeric: Anti-inflammatory spice that supports thyroid function.

17. Ginger : Promotes digestion and aids in nutrient absorption.

18. Sea Salt: Contains iodine, essential for thyroid hormone synthesis.

19. Apple Cider Vinegar: Supports digestion and may help balance blood sugar levels.

20. Fresh Herbs: Parsley, cilantro, basil – add flavor and micronutrients to your dishes.

Miscellaneous

21. Seaweed: A natural source of iodine, crucial for thyroid hormone synthesis.

22. Coconut Oil: Contains medium-chain fatty acids that support metabolism.

23. Dark Chocolate: In moderation, provides antioxidants and may boost mood.

24. Green Tea: Rich in antioxidants and may support weight management.

25. Bone Broth: Contains collagen and amino acids that promote gut health and immunity.

Advice

- **Variety is Key:** Aim for a diverse range of foods to ensure you're obtaining all the necessary nutrients.
- **Read Labels:** Be mindful of added sugars, preservatives, and artificial ingredients in packaged foods.
- **Stay Hydrated:** Drink plenty of water throughout the day to support metabolism and overall health.
- **Listen to Your Body:** Pay attention to how different foods make you feel and adjust your diet accordingly.
- **Consult a Professional:** Consider working with a registered dietitian or nutritionist to tailor a plan that suits your individual needs and goals.

As you embark on this journey, remember that nourishing your body is a form of self-care and empowerment. With each mindful choice you make, you are nurturing your thyroid and fostering a deeper connection with your own well-being. Embrace the journey, savor the flavors, and revel in the vitality that awaits you.

Monitoring Development and Adapting for Achievement

It is advised to keep a daily journal to make monitoring improvement easier. This includes keeping track of your meals, energy levels, and any noteworthy thyroid-related symptoms. Weekly reflections give people the chance to evaluate changes in their general well-being, energy levels, and emotional state.

To give objective statistics on success, the meal plan recommends periodic thyroid function testing in addition to self-monitoring. The meal plan can be modified to suit each person's requirements based on the outcomes. This adaptability guarantees that the strategy may be modified to meet changing health needs, promoting a long-term, sustainable approach to thyroid health. Frequent evaluations and modifications are part of a comprehensive and individualized plan for enhancing thyroid function and general health.